Revolutionizing Migraine Therapy with Lu AG09222

Table of Content

Abstract 3

Migraine 4

Migraine triggers 4

Phases...........4

Introduction .5

Pathophysiology of migraine 7

Role of PACAP 10

Lu AG09222 12

Moa of Lu AG09222   13

Clinical trial.14

Difference between Lu AG09222 and other therapies for Migraine   16

Conclusion ..19

Abbreviations 21

Abstract

Migraine is a widespread and enfeebling common headache illness that is frequently misunderstood and underdiagnosed. It is distinguished by throbbing, unilateral pain, which is usually accompanied by nausea, reactive to bright light and loud sound, and worsens with frequent motion. If left untreated, migraine attacks can persist for a long time from 4 to 72 hours. Migraines are a neurovascular illness characterized by blood vessel dilatation and nerve activation. Peptides such as PACAP and VIP have an important part in migraine pathogenesis, with PACAP known to cause migraine attacks. In this review we will discuss about an emerging drug which is a monoclonal antibody, Lu AG09222 and is now being developed (phase III) to target PACAP for migraine prevention and can present a novel and enhanced option to cure the migraine.

Keyword – Migraine, Headache, PACAP, Lu AG09222

Migraine

A migraine is a severe headache that causes throbbing, pulsing head pain on one side of your head. The headache phase of a migraine usually lasts at least four hours, but it can also last for days. This headache gets worse with: Physical activity.

Migraine triggers

- Disturbed sleep pattern
- Hormonal changes
- Drugs
- Physical exertion
- Visual stimuli
- Auditory stimuli
- Hunger

- Psychological factors

Phases

There are four phases in migraine

- Prodrome
- Aura
- Headache
- Postdrome

Introduction

Headache are one of the common and most prevalent types of recurring discomfort, and very frequently discussed complaints in neurology and Headache diseases are classified mainly into Primary and Secondary categories. Secondary Migraine Headaches have a clear underlying reason, such as brain tumor, infection, or stroke and Primary migraine headache shows no clear underlying etiology. One of the most problematic primary headache diseases is migraine, which is still poorly recognized, underdiagnosed, and undertreated in professional area and it is an intricate neurological condition that has been identified since ancient times. The primary symptoms of a migraine are a throbbing, frequently unilateral headache, along with accompanying symptoms like light and sound sensitivity, nausea, and worsening with head movement. When left untreated, these attacks typically last 4 to 72 hours. Migraine is a type of neurovascular headache: a condition in which neuronal events cause the expansion of the blood vessels, which results in pain and additional neurostimulation. Vasoactive intestinal peptide (VIP) and pituitary adenylate cyclase-activating polypeptide (PACAP) are important migraine triggers. They have a lot in common and belong to the same structurally related vasoactive peptide superfamily, glucagon/secretin. PACAP belongs to the VIP/secretin/glucagon neuropeptide family and exists in two physiologically active forms: PACAP27 and mostly PACAP38 and this is a pleiotropic peptide that serves as a hormone of the pituitary gland, a neurotransmitter, and a neuromodulator in the nervous system, while also exhibiting anti-apoptotic, neuroprotective & differentiation-inducing characteristics in the developing nervous system. PACAP exerts its effects through G-protein-coupled receptors: PAC 1, VPAC 2, and VPAC 1 [8] and in the humans, PACAP38 causes dilation of extracerebral arteries, triggers headaches in healthy persons, and precipitates migraine episodes in those with a history of migraines. For the treatment of migraine an experimental humanized monoclonal antibody targeting PACAP, known as Lu AG09222, is presently undergoing development for the prevention of migraines. Lu AG09222 attaches to PACAP and blocks receptor binding. Although it is still in the trial phase, if successful, Lu AG09222 has the potential to become a pioneering treatment focusing on a new pathway for preventing migraines.

Pathophysiology of migraine

The Trigeminovascular (TVS) system, having the trigeminal nerve and the vascular connections, is critical to the pathogenesis of migraine. Activation of this system causes the secretion of vasoactive neuropeptides, such as calcitonin gene-related peptide (CGRP), substance P, and neurokinin A, which induce vasodilation and neurogenic inflammation within the meninges. In Migraine CGRP, in particular, has been intensively investigated and recognized as a significant mediator of migraine pain, prompting the development of CGRP-targeted treatments, such as monoclonal antibodies and receptor antagonists. The neuroinflammatory process involves the activation of glial cells and the secretion of pro-inflammatory cytokines, which exacerbate pain transmission and contribute to central sensitization. Central sensitization is a phenomenon where repeated activation of trigeminal pathways enhances the excitability of central neurons, making them more responsive to pain stimuli and contributing to the persistence of headache and the development of allodynia. The role of serotonin in migraine pathophysiology is also significant, with fluctuations in serotonin levels affecting vascular tone and trigeminal system activity. Serotonin 5-HT1B/1D receptor agonists, such as triptans, are very effective in acute migraine treatment by inhibiting the release of CGRP and inducing vasoconstriction. Moreover, neuroimaging studies shows abnormal activation patterns in the hypothalamus, brainstem, and other cortical areas during migraine attacks, suggesting a broader network dysfunction beyond the trigeminovascular system. The hypothalamus, in particular, is implicated in the premonitory symptoms of migraine, such as fatigue, mood changes, and food cravings, which takes place hours to days before the headache phase. Migraine pathophysiology also involves a dysregulation of the autonomic nervous system, which may explain the linked symptoms such as nausea, vomiting & photophobia. Functional imaging has revealed hyperactivity in brain regions responsible for autonomic control during migraine attacks Additionally, hormonal fluctuations, particularly those related to estrogen, are known to influence migraine susceptibility, explaining the increased prevalence of migraine in women and its association with the menstrual cycle. Finally, ongoing research into the role of oxidative stress, mitochondrial dysfunction, and cortical excitability continues to shed light on the complex mechanisms underlying this debilitating disorder. PACAP also plays a very important part in the Migraine pathophysiology which has been discussed below.

Role of PACAP

There is a substantial correlation between PACAP and the pathophysiology of migraine. The trigeminal nerve, believed to be crucial in this illness, has high amounts of PACAP. It is well established that PACAP causes inflammation, dilatation of brain blood vessels, and increase in the sensitivity of trigeminal nerve. The onset of migraine episodes has been linked to each of these physiologic processes. Numerous research endeavors have been carried out to examine the function of PACAP in migraine. According to one study, blood levels of PACAP are considerably greater in migraine sufferers during an episode than in controls who do not have a headache. Numerous research endeavors have been carried out to examine the function of PACAP in migraine. According to one study, blood levels of PACAP are considerably greater in migraine sufferers during an episode than in people without headaches. According to this study,

PACAP may be a useful biomarker for migraine. Another study showed that migraine patients who received venous infusions of PACAP developed migraine-like symptoms. Numerous studies provide compelling evidence in favor of the theory that PACAP is one of the important factors in the migraine pathophysiology and raise the possibility of using PACAP inhibition as a therapeutic target to treat migraines. There is substantial evidence to support the well-established involvement of PACAP in pathophysiology of migraine, including its critical role in the onset of migraine episodes. To create novel pharmaceutical compounds that target PACAP and treat migraines, further study and research is required to comprehend the mechanism of action of PACAP.

Lu AG09222

Lu AG09222 is an investigational monoclonal antibody being developed by Lundbeck as a potential preventive treatment for migraines. It specifically targets and inhibits the signaling of PACAP, a neuropeptide involved in the pathophysiology of migraine. This makes Lu AG09222 distinct from current migraine treatments from those which typically targets CGRP pathways. "Lu AG09222 is novel because it targets the PACAP ligand itself, rather than specific PACAP receptors, "This approach avoids the complexities of identifying which PACAP receptors are involved in migraine, offering a potentially more direct and effective mechanism for treatment." Lu AG09222 is currently in Phase III clinical trials managed by Lundbeck and if successful it will become a novel treatment to treat migraine.

Moa of Lu AG09222

A Monoclonal antibody Lu AG09222 which is designed to target and stop or inhibit the activity of PACAP, a neuropeptide involved in the pathophysiology of migraines. As we know PACAP is a neuropeptide which plays a significant part in the development and propagation of migraine attacks it induces vasodilation and activates the pain pathway in the brain and contribute to the migraine symptom. When administered Lu AG09222 it works by binding to PACAP with high affinity, effectively neutralizing its ability to interact with its receptors. This prevents PACAP from triggering the cascade of biological processes that lead to migraine headaches, such as vasodilation and activation of pain receptors since migraine attacks are often linked to the changes of blood flow in the brain

Clinical trial

There are some studies which have shown a great result in the development of treatment for migraine and one of the recent trials which was conducted at Danish Headache Center, Glostrup Hospital, University Hospital Copenhagen, Denmark to check the potency of Lu AG09222. It is a randomized, double-blind, parallel-group single-dose placebo-controlled study at the Danish Headache Center, Glostrup Hospital, University Hospital Copenhagen, Denmark, healthy volunteers (18-45 years of age) with history of headache conditions were chosen at random and assigned to one of three treatment sequences (1:2:2) for two experimental infusion visits 9±3 days apart. The major outcome measure was the AUC for change in STA diameter from 0 to 120 minutes after starting PACAP38 infusion. Subjects who received Lu AG09222 in conjunction with PACAP38 had a substantially reduced STA diameter (mean (SE) [95% CI] AUC −35.4 (4.32) [−44.6, −26.3] mm × min; $P < 0.0001$) than those who received (placebo + PACAP38). This suggests that Lu AG09222 may be a possible therapeutic for migraines and other PACAP-mediated disorders.

In the trial, subjects were divided into three groups as shown in Table 1: the Placebo + Saline + Saline group (n=5), the Placebo + PACAP38 + VIP group (n=10), and the

LuAG09222 + PACAP38 + VIP group (n=10). The results of the trial, presented in Table 2, indicate that in the Placebo + PACAP38 + VIP group, PACAP38 administration resulted in an increase in superficial temporal artery (STA) diameter. Additionally, PACAP38 was found to increase facial blood flow, heart rate, and cause a moderate headache. Conversely, in the LuAG09222 + PACAP38 + VIP group, LuAG09222 significantly reduced the STA diameter. It also mitigated the PACAP38-induced increases in facial blood flow, heart rate, and moderate headache, showing a potential therapeutic effect

Difference between Lu AG09222 and other therapies for Migraine

Lu AG09222 is a monoclonal antibody targeting the pituitary adenylate cyclase-activating polypeptide (PACAP), a neuropeptide involved in the pathophysiology of migraines. By inhibiting PACAP, Lu AG09222 aims to block an upstream mediator of migraine attacks without causing vasoconstriction, offering a targeted approach to migraine prevention. This contrasts with treatments targeting calcitonin gene-related peptide (CGRP) or its receptor, such as CGRP monoclonal antibodies (erenumab, fremanezumab, and galcanezumab), which block CGRP, a neuropeptide that promotes vasodilation and transmits pain signals. Gepants (e.g., rimegepant, ubrogepant) also target the CGRP receptor, but they are oral medications used for both acute treatment and prevention, acting by preventing CGRP from binding to its receptor during migraine attacks.

Unlike Lu AG09222, which works through PACAP inhibition, triptans (e.g., sumatriptan, rizatriptan, zolmitriptan) are 5-HT1B/1D receptor agonists used primarily for acute migraine relief. These medications cause vasoconstriction by preventing the release of pro-inflammatory neuropeptides like CGRP, effectively reducing migraine symptoms during an attack. While effective for acute relief, triptans act on a broader scale and are not typically used for prevention.

Other treatments like nonsteroidal anti-inflammatory drugs (NSAIDs) and analgesics focus on relieving symptoms such as pain and inflammation without specifically targeting the migraine pathways. Similarly, botulinum toxin

(Botox) is used for chronic migraine prevention by inhibiting acetylcholine release at neuromuscular junctions, reducing muscle contractions and preventing pain pathway activation. Though effective in chronic cases, these treatments do not directly inhibit neuropeptides involved in migraine pathogenesis, making them less targeted than monoclonal antibody therapies like Lu AG09222.

Overall, Lu AG09222 offers a more precise approach by targeting PACAP, potentially providing relief from migraines without the vascular side effects of other treatments. Like other monoclonal antibodies, it is likely administered via injection.

Conclusion

As we conclude our discussion, we have come to conclude that Migraine is a prevalent and enfeebling neurovascular condition Distinguished by strong, frequent one-sided, pulsating headaches, queasiness, sensitivity to light and sound, and, in some instances, vomiting. If left untreated, these episodes can persist for anywhere from (4 to 72 hours). Even though they are very common, migraine is frequently not diagnosed and inadequately treated in clinical settings. Its underlying cause is intricate, primarily involving the TVS system. The activation of the trigeminal nerve and the blood arteries that supply it cause the production of neuropeptides such as neurokinin A, substance P & CGRP. These neuropeptides show vasodilation and neurogenic inflammation, which exacerbates the pain associated with migraine episodes. PACAP, a neuropeptide abundant in the trigeminal system, plays a significant role in migraine pathophysiology. PACAP has been shown to trigger migraine-like attacks by increasing vasodilation, trigeminal nerve sensitivity, and inflammation. Its importance in migraine has made it a compelling target for therapy. Research has shown heightened PACAP levels during migraine attacks, and its administration in individuals has resulted in migraine onset, further confirming its involvement. One of the most promising advancements in migraine treatment is the monoclonal antibody Lu AG09222, which is currently undergoing advanced clinical trials. Lu AG09222 aims to selectively bind to and neutralize PACAP, preventing it from binding to its receptors and thereby disrupting the series of circumstances that result in migraine. Unlike current migraine medications, which primarily target CGRP, Lu AG09222 offers a different approach by focusing on PACAP, a neuropeptide upstream in the migraine pathway. If successful, Lu AG09222 could become a pioneering medication, offering a new option for migraine prevention that does not rely on vasoconstriction, a common mechanism in many existing treatments. This could represent a significant breakthrough, delivering relief to the millions of individuals suffering from this debilitating condition.

Abbreviations

PACAP – Pituitary adenylate cyclase-activating polypeptide

VIP – vasoactive intestinal peptide

CGRP – calcitonin gene-related peptide

5-HT1B/1D – Triptans

TVS – Trigeminovascular system

STA – Superficial temporal artery

AUC – Area under curve

www.ingramcontent.com/pod-product-compliance
Lightning Source LLC
Chambersburg PA
CBHW071001220526
45471CB00007B/3121